Brain Longevity & Cognitive Youth

Advanced Strategies to Preserve Memory, Focus, and Mental Sharpness for Life

By Joe Correa

Published by Live Stronger Faster

This book is for educational and informational purposes only. The author and publisher are not engaged in rendering legal, financial, or other professional advice. Readers should consult a qualified professional before making any financial decisions.

First Edition

Table of Contents

Introduction

The human brain is the most complex biological system ever discovered, yet it is also one of the most vulnerable to the effects of aging. While wrinkles, joint stiffness, and reduced muscle mass are often accepted as visible signs of aging, cognitive decline is far more feared—and for good reason. Memory loss, reduced focus, slower processing speed, emotional instability, and neurodegenerative disease threaten not only lifespan, but identity, independence, and quality of life itself. Brain longevity is therefore not optional. It is central to true longevity.

For decades, brain aging was viewed as inevitable: neurons die, synapses weaken, cognition fades, and decline accelerates with time. Modern neuroscience has proven this assumption wrong. The brain is not a static organ destined for decay—it is dynamic, adaptive, and remarkably capable of renewal when the correct biological conditions are present. Neuroplasticity, neurogenesis, synaptic remodeling, and metabolic flexibility allow the brain to remain youthful well into advanced age, provided it is properly supported.

This book exists to teach you how to create those conditions deliberately. Brain longevity is not achieved through crossword puzzles alone, nor is it preserved by supplements in isolation. It requires a systems-based approach that integrates metabolism, inflammation control, mitochondrial function, vascular health, sleep architecture, stress regulation, nutrition, movement, hormonal balance, and cognitive stimulation. Every chapter of this book builds upon the foundation laid across the previous volumes in this series, translating whole-body longevity principles into precise strategies for cognitive preservation.

By the end of this book, you will understand not only how the brain ages, but why it ages—and more importantly, how to slow, halt, and in some cases reverse key mechanisms of cognitive decline.

The Brain as a Longevity Bottleneck

Longevity without cognitive health is not success—it is survival. A long life with a failing mind places an enormous burden on individuals, families, and healthcare systems. Dementia, Alzheimer's disease, Parkinson's disease, and age-related cognitive impairment represent some of the fastest-growing medical challenges worldwide. Yet many of these conditions are not purely genetic or random; they are the cumulative result of decades of metabolic stress, inflammation, vascular damage, nutrient deficiencies, hormonal dysregulation, and nervous system overload. The brain consumes approximately 20% of the body's total energy while accounting for only 2% of its weight. This makes it exquisitely sensitive to mitochondrial dysfunction, insulin resistance, poor blood flow, and oxidative stress. When energy production falters, cognition is among the first systems to suffer. Brain fog, attention problems, mood instability, and memory lapses are early warning signs—not inconveniences.

This book reframes brain decline as a **process**, not an event. Just as cardiovascular disease develops silently for years before a heart attack, cognitive decline begins decades before diagnosis. The strategies in this book are designed to intervene early, reinforce resilience, and extend cognitive youth across the entire lifespan.

Cognitive Youth Is a Trainable State

One of the most empowering discoveries in neuroscience is that cognitive youth is not fixed—it is trainable. Learning new skills, challenging existing neural pathways, optimizing metabolic fuel sources, and regulating the stress response all contribute to sustained neuroplasticity. The brain remodels itself in response to inputs, both positive and negative.

This book will teach you how to:

- Preserve and enhance memory formation and recall

- Maintain executive function, decision-making, and mental clarity
- Protect neurons from inflammation, oxidative stress, and metabolic damage
- Improve attention span and cognitive endurance
- Support emotional regulation and mental resilience
- Reduce long-term risk of neurodegenerative disease

These outcomes are not achieved through mental stimulation alone. They require biological alignment. Cognitive performance is inseparable from sleep quality, insulin sensitivity, cardiovascular health, gut integrity, hormonal balance, and nervous system tone. Brain longevity is a **whole-body project**, and this book integrates each system into a cohesive strategy.

Why Brain Aging Accelerates in Modern Life

Modern environments are hostile to brain longevity. Chronic stress, sleep deprivation, ultra-processed diets, sedentary behavior, excessive screen exposure, constant dopamine stimulation, and environmental toxins all place sustained pressure on the nervous system. The result is accelerated neural aging, even in younger populations.

Key contributors to accelerated brain aging include:

- Chronic low-grade inflammation
- Insulin resistance and glucose volatility
- Poor sleep architecture and circadian disruption
- Mitochondrial dysfunction
- Reduced cerebral blood flow
- Excess cortisol and sympathetic nervous system dominance
- Lack of cognitive novelty and challenge

This book does not merely identify these factors—it provides actionable methods to counteract them. You will learn how to create a brain-supportive environment through daily routines, nutritional strategies, movement protocols, recovery practices, and cognitive training that reinforce neural resilience.

The Brain–Body Connection in Longevity

The brain does not age in isolation. It reflects the state of the entire organism. Poor metabolic health accelerates brain aging. Chronic inflammation damages neural tissue. Hormonal imbalance disrupts neurotransmitter signaling.

Sleep deprivation impairs memory consolidation. Gut dysfunction alters mood and cognition through the gut-brain axis. This is why brain longevity cannot be separated from the principles covered in earlier books in this series. Cellular rejuvenation, mitochondrial efficiency, inflammation control, epigenetic regulation, nutrition timing, and nervous system recovery all converge in the brain.

In this book, you will learn how to integrate these systems specifically for cognitive outcomes. The strategies presented here are designed to be layered on top of your existing longevity framework, creating a synergistic effect that amplifies results across both mental and physical domains.

From Cognitive Decline to Cognitive Expansion

Brain longevity is not merely about prevention—it is about expansion. Many individuals experience improved memory, sharper focus, faster learning, and greater emotional stability well into midlife and beyond when the correct protocols are applied. Aging does not require mental contraction. In fact, certain cognitive abilities—including pattern recognition, wisdom, emotional intelligence, and strategic thinking—can improve with age when the brain is properly supported.

This book emphasizes proactive cognitive expansion rather than defensive decline management. You will be guided to build cognitive reserve, strengthen neural networks, and enhance mental adaptability so that your brain remains capable, curious, and engaged throughout life.

What This Book Will Teach You

Throughout this book, you will learn:

- How memory is formed, stored, and retrieved—and how to protect these processes
- How insulin resistance and metabolic dysfunction affect cognition
- How sleep architecture supports memory consolidation and emotional regulation
- How stress hormones accelerate brain aging and how to rebalance them
- How inflammation damages neural tissue and how to reduce it systemically
- How movement, blood flow, and oxygenation preserve cognitive performance
- How to create daily brain longevity routines that compound over time

Each chapter builds logically, moving from foundational neuroscience principles to advanced, actionable strategies that can be implemented immediately.

Brain Longevity as a Lifelong Investment

Cognitive youth is one of the highest-return investments you can make. Unlike material assets, mental clarity compounds across every domain of life—career performance, relationships, creativity, decision-making, emotional stability, and independence. Protecting your brain is not an act of fear; it is an act of strategy.

This book invites you to take ownership of your cognitive future. Brain longevity is not reserved for the genetically lucky or the medically privileged. It is the result of informed, consistent choices made over time. The strategies within these pages are designed to empower you with knowledge, clarity, and control.

As you move into the chapters ahead, approach this book not as passive reading, but as a blueprint. Your brain is adaptable. Your cognitive future is not predetermined. And with the right systems in place, mental sharpness can remain one of your greatest assets for life.

Chapter 1

The Aging Brain: What Really Happens Over Time

The aging of the brain is often misunderstood as a sudden decline rather than a slow, cumulative biological process. In reality, brain aging begins quietly, sometimes as early as the third decade of life, shaped by metabolic health, inflammation levels, sleep quality, stress exposure, and environmental inputs. The brain does not simply "wear out." It adapts to conditions—good or bad—and its structure, chemistry, and performance reflect the environment it is forced to operate within. Understanding this process is the first step toward preserving cognitive youth.

At a structural level, the aging brain experiences changes in synaptic density, neurotransmitter production, cerebral blood flow, and mitochondrial efficiency. Neurons themselves may survive for decades, but the connections between them—the synapses—can weaken or disappear if not regularly reinforced. These synaptic changes directly affect memory formation, processing speed, attention, and emotional regulation. Cognitive decline, therefore, is less about neuron loss and more about network degradation. One of the earliest drivers of brain aging is metabolic dysfunction. The brain relies heavily on glucose and oxygen to fuel neuronal activity. When insulin resistance develops, glucose uptake in the brain becomes inefficient, leading to energy deficits that impair cognition. This metabolic stress contributes to brain fog, memory lapses, and reduced mental stamina. Over time, chronic energy deprivation accelerates neuronal vulnerability and synaptic loss.

Inflammation is another major contributor to brain aging. While acute inflammation is a protective response, chronic low-grade inflammation—often driven by poor diet, stress, gut dysfunction, and sedentary behavior—creates a hostile environment for neural tissue. Inflammatory cytokines interfere with neurotransmitter signaling, damage blood-brain barrier integrity, and impair neuroplasticity. The result is a brain that becomes less adaptable and more prone to degeneration.

Mitochondrial decline plays a central role in this process. Neurons are among the most energy-dependent cells in the body, and their mitochondria must function efficiently to sustain cognitive performance. As mitochondrial efficiency decreases with age, neurons struggle to maintain electrical signaling and synaptic communication. This energy shortfall contributes not only to cognitive slowing but also to increased susceptibility to neurodegenerative disease. Cerebral blood flow also declines with age, particularly in individuals with cardiovascular risk factors such as hypertension, atherosclerosis, and poor endothelial function. Reduced blood flow limits oxygen and nutrient delivery to the brain, impairing memory, focus, and executive function. This vascular component of brain aging is often overlooked, yet it is one of the most modifiable risk factors for cognitive decline.

Hormonal changes further influence brain aging. Declines in estrogen, testosterone, growth hormone, and DHEA affect neurotransmitter balance, neuroprotection, and synaptic plasticity. Cortisol, the primary stress hormone, often increases with age due to chronic stress exposure. Elevated cortisol damages the hippocampus, the brain region responsible for memory and learning, accelerating cognitive decline when left unchecked.

Sleep disruption is another powerful accelerator of brain aging. During deep sleep, the brain clears metabolic waste, consolidates memory, and repairs neural tissue. Chronic sleep deprivation or poor sleep architecture interferes with these processes, leading to toxin accumulation, impaired memory consolidation, and emotional instability. Over time, insufficient sleep creates a compounding deficit that accelerates cognitive aging. Importantly, brain aging is not uniform across individuals. Lifestyle choices exert enormous influence over the rate and severity of cognitive decline. Diet quality, physical activity, cognitive engagement, stress management, and social connection all shape neural health. The brain continuously remodels itself in response to these inputs, meaning decline is not inevitable—it is conditional.

Neuroplasticity remains present throughout life, although it becomes more dependent on deliberate stimulation with age. Learning new skills, engaging in complex problem-solving, and exposing the brain to novelty stimulate synaptic growth and network resilience. Without these challenges, neural pathways weaken through disuse, reinforcing patterns of decline.

This chapter establishes a critical truth: brain aging is a process that can be influenced, slowed, and partially reversed. Cognitive youth is not a genetic accident—it is a biological outcome shaped by daily inputs. The chapters that follow will build on this foundation, translating neuroscience into practical strategies that preserve mental sharpness and protect the brain for life.

Daniel had always been sharp

Daniel noticed the change long before anyone else did. It wasn't dramatic or sudden. It was subtle—names that lingered just out of reach, conversations that felt harder to follow, a sense that his thoughts no longer moved with the same effortless clarity they once had. At fifty-six, he told himself it was normal. Everyone forgot things. Everyone slowed down. That was just aging, wasn't it?

Yet deep down, he felt unsettled. Daniel had always been sharp. He built a career on quick thinking, strategic insight, and mental endurance. Now, after long days, his mind felt foggy instead of fulfilled. Evenings that once sparked creativity were replaced by mental exhaustion. He began to wonder whether this was simply the price of time—or a warning.

One afternoon, after struggling to recall a colleague's name mid-conversation, Daniel felt something shift. Not panic, but resolve. He realized that physical aging had always seemed manageable—exercise, nutrition, discipline. But mental aging had gone unquestioned. He had never been taught how to protect his brain.

As Daniel began learning about how the brain actually ages, a quiet sense of relief emerged. His symptoms weren't random. They had explanations. Years of chronic stress, poor sleep, rushed meals, and sedentary habits had shaped his brain just as surely as they had shaped his body. The realization was empowering. If decline was learned, then resilience could be rebuilt.

He started small. Improving sleep. Walking daily. Challenging his brain with learning instead of passive entertainment. Over weeks, something remarkable happened. The fog lifted. His thoughts felt more fluid. Conversations energized him again. His memory sharpened—not perfectly, but noticeably.

Months later, Daniel noticed something else. He felt mentally younger than he had a decade earlier. Not reckless or naive, but clear, focused, and emotionally steady. The fear he once carried about aging had been replaced by confidence. His brain wasn't fading—it was adapting.

Daniel's story is not extraordinary because of who he is, but because of what it reveals. Cognitive decline is not an unavoidable fate. It is often a signal—an invitation to change the conditions the brain lives in. When those conditions improve, the brain responds.

This book exists for people like Daniel. People who refuse to accept mental decline as inevitable. People who believe that clarity, curiosity, and sharp thinking should not disappear with age. Brain longevity is not about resisting time—it is about partnering with biology.

Your brain is listening to how you live. Every choice you make sends a signal. This chapter marks the beginning of a new conversation with your mind—one grounded in science, intention, and possibility. Cognitive youth is not behind you. With the right systems in place, it can remain with you for life.

Chapter 2

Neuroplasticity: How the Brain Stays Young by Rebuilding Itself

Neuroplasticity is the brain's fundamental mechanism for adaptation, learning, and renewal. It refers to the brain's ability to reorganize neural networks by forming new synaptic connections in response to experience, learning, injury, and environmental input. Contrary to outdated beliefs, neuroplasticity does not end in childhood. While its speed and intensity may decline with age, the capacity for neural remodeling remains present throughout life when properly stimulated and supported.

At its core, neuroplasticity is driven by use. Neural circuits that are frequently activated become stronger, faster, and more efficient, while those that are neglected weaken and eventually disappear through a process known as synaptic pruning. This biological efficiency allows the brain to conserve energy, but it also means that passivity accelerates decline. Cognitive youth depends on continual engagement, novelty, and challenge.

Learning is one of the most powerful stimulators of neuroplasticity. When the brain encounters unfamiliar information or tasks, it is forced to build new neural pathways.

This process increases synaptic density, enhances communication between brain regions, and improves cognitive flexibility. Importantly, learning does not need to be academic. New physical skills, languages, instruments, strategic games, and problem-solving tasks all stimulate neuroplastic change.

Movement also plays a critical role in neural remodeling. Physical activity increases blood flow to the brain, enhances oxygen and nutrient delivery, and stimulates the release of neurotrophic factors that support neuron survival and growth. Regular movement improves coordination between the motor cortex, cerebellum, and executive centers, reinforcing whole-brain integration. Sedentary behavior, by contrast, deprives the brain of essential stimulation and accelerates neural decline.

Sleep is another essential driver of neuroplasticity. During deep sleep, the brain consolidates learning by strengthening newly formed synapses and pruning inefficient connections. Memory integration, emotional processing, and neural repair occur most effectively during high-quality sleep cycles. Chronic sleep disruption interferes with these processes, reducing the brain's ability to adapt and recover.

Stress has a profound influence on neuroplastic capacity. Short-term stress can enhance learning and alertness, but chronic stress suppresses neuroplasticity by elevating cortisol levels. Excess cortisol damages the hippocampus, impairs memory formation, and reduces synaptic growth. Stress management is therefore not optional for cognitive longevity—it is foundational.

Nutrition supports neuroplasticity through its effects on inflammation, mitochondrial function, and neurotransmitter synthesis. Adequate protein intake supplies amino acids necessary for neurotransmitter production, while healthy fats support myelin integrity and synaptic signaling. Micronutrients such as magnesium, zinc, and B vitamins play critical roles in neural communication. Nutritional deficiencies silently impair plasticity long before cognitive symptoms appear.

Social interaction is an often-overlooked driver of neuroplasticity. Meaningful social engagement challenges emotional regulation, language processing, memory recall, and executive function simultaneously. Isolation reduces neural stimulation across multiple brain regions, accelerating decline. Longevity research consistently shows that socially connected individuals preserve cognitive function longer than those who are isolated.

Importantly, neuroplasticity is directionally neutral. The brain adapts to what it repeatedly experiences. Negative patterns—rumination, chronic anxiety, multitasking, and overstimulation—can strengthen maladaptive neural circuits just as easily as positive ones. Intentionality matters. Cognitive youth requires deliberate cultivation of adaptive patterns.

Neuroplasticity also underlies recovery. Even after injury or decline, the brain can reroute functions through alternative pathways. This capacity is strongest when the brain is metabolically healthy, well-rested, emotionally regulated, and adequately stimulated. Aging does not eliminate plasticity—it raises the threshold required to activate it.

This chapter establishes neuroplasticity as the central mechanism of brain longevity. Cognitive youth is not maintained by preservation alone, but by continuous renewal. The chapters that follow will build upon this principle, translating plasticity into targeted strategies for memory, focus, emotional stability, and long-term cognitive resilience.

Maria didn't know the term neuroplasticity

Maria never thought of herself as someone who could change her brain. At sixty-two, she believed that who she was—how she thought, what she remembered, how quickly she learned—was already decided. She had accepted the narrative that aging meant narrowing: fewer new skills, fewer new ideas, fewer surprises.

Her days had become predictable. Familiar routines, familiar conversations, familiar thoughts. Comfortable, but quiet. Over time, she noticed her world shrinking—not physically, but mentally. She felt less curious, less confident trying new things. It wasn't sadness exactly, more like dullness.

Everything shifted when her granddaughter asked her to learn a new game together. Maria hesitated, embarrassed by how hard it felt to follow unfamiliar rules. But she agreed. The first few sessions were frustrating. She forgot steps, repeated mistakes, and felt slow. Yet something unexpected happened. She felt alive.

As weeks passed, the fog she had accepted as "normal" began to lift. Her focus sharpened. She started remembering details more easily. Encouraged, Maria tried something else—learning a new recipe, walking a different route, reading topics she had never explored before. Each challenge felt uncomfortable at first, but satisfying afterward.

Maria didn't know the term neuroplasticity, but she was living it. Her brain was responding to novelty, effort, and engagement. Old assumptions about limitation began to dissolve. She realized her brain wasn't closed—it had simply been underused.

One afternoon, she caught herself laughing at how different she felt. Not younger in age, but lighter in mind. More flexible. More capable. The world felt larger again. Possibility had returned. Maria's transformation wasn't dramatic from the outside. But internally, it was profound. She had proven to herself that growth didn't end with age—it required intention. The brain, she learned, listens closely to how it is treated.

Her story reflects a truth available to everyone. Cognitive youth is not a memory—it is a practice. Every new challenge is a signal to the brain that growth is still required. Every moment of curiosity is an invitation for renewal.

This chapter is a reminder that your brain is not finished evolving. No matter your age, it is still learning from you. What you choose to repeat, what you choose to avoid, and what you choose to explore will shape your cognitive future.

Neuroplasticity is not about becoming someone else. It is about becoming more of who you already are—clearer, sharper, and more alive. And that process can begin at any moment you decide to challenge your mind again.

Chapter 3

Brain Fuel & Metabolic Intelligence: How Energy Determines Cognitive Lifespan

The brain is not limited by intelligence alone; it is constrained by energy. Every thought, memory, emotion, and decision is powered by metabolic processes that determine how efficiently neurons communicate. Cognitive decline is often framed as a neurological issue, but at its foundation, it is frequently a metabolic one. When the brain's energy systems falter, mental performance follows.

The brain requires a constant supply of fuel to maintain electrical signaling, neurotransmitter production, and synaptic communication. Although it represents only a small fraction of total body mass, it consumes a disproportionate share of energy. This makes the brain uniquely sensitive to fluctuations in blood sugar, insulin signaling, oxygen availability, and mitochondrial efficiency. Stability, not abundance, is the key to cognitive longevity.

Glucose has long been considered the brain's primary fuel source, but modern research reveals a more nuanced picture. While glucose is essential, chronic glucose spikes followed by crashes create metabolic stress that impairs cognitive function. Repeated blood sugar volatility damages neurons, increases inflammation, and accelerates insulin resistance in the brain itself. Over time, this leads to a condition sometimes referred to as "type 3 diabetes," where the brain becomes less responsive to insulin and less capable of efficiently using glucose for energy.

Insulin resistance in the brain disrupts memory formation, learning capacity, and executive function. Neurons struggle to absorb glucose, leading to energy deficits that manifest as brain fog, mental fatigue, and slowed cognition. This metabolic impairment often precedes noticeable cognitive decline by years, making it a critical early intervention point for brain longevity.

Mitochondria serve as the cellular engines that convert fuel into usable energy. In neurons, mitochondrial efficiency determines the brain's capacity for sustained focus, rapid processing, and emotional regulation. As mitochondrial function declines with age, neurons become more vulnerable to oxidative stress and energy failure. Supporting mitochondrial health is therefore central to preserving cognitive youth.

Alternative fuel sources, such as ketones, offer a powerful metabolic advantage for the aging brain. Ketones provide a stable, efficient energy source that bypasses some of the insulin-related limitations of glucose metabolism. When available, ketones reduce oxidative stress, improve mitochondrial efficiency, and enhance neuronal resilience. This metabolic flexibility becomes increasingly valuable as glucose tolerance declines with age.

Inflammation further complicates brain energy metabolism. Chronic inflammation interferes with insulin signaling, damages mitochondrial membranes, and disrupts neurotransmitter balance. Inflammatory pathways divert energy away from cognitive function toward immune response, creating a persistent energy deficit in the brain. Reducing systemic inflammation restores metabolic efficiency and supports long-term cognitive performance.

Blood flow and oxygen delivery are also critical determinants of brain energy availability. Neurons require oxygen to generate ATP efficiently. Reduced cerebral blood flow, often associated with cardiovascular disease, sedentary behavior, and endothelial dysfunction, limits oxygen delivery and impairs cognitive function. Enhancing vascular health directly supports brain metabolism and longevity.

Micronutrients play an essential role in energy production. Magnesium supports ATP synthesis, B vitamins facilitate glucose and fat metabolism, iron supports oxygen transport, and antioxidants protect mitochondria from oxidative damage. Even mild deficiencies can significantly impair brain energy systems, highlighting the importance of nutrient sufficiency for cognitive health.

Energy metabolism also influences neurotransmitter balance. The synthesis and recycling of dopamine, serotonin, acetylcholine, and GABA all depend on adequate energy availability. When fuel supply is inconsistent or inefficient, neurotransmitter production suffers, leading to mood instability, reduced motivation, impaired memory, and diminished focus.

Cognitive endurance—the ability to think clearly for extended periods—is a direct reflection of metabolic resilience. Brains with stable fuel access and efficient mitochondria sustain attention, resist fatigue, and recover quickly from mental exertion. Those operating under metabolic stress experience rapid exhaustion and cognitive decline under pressure.

This chapter establishes a foundational principle: brain longevity depends on metabolic intelligence. By stabilizing fuel supply, enhancing mitochondrial efficiency, reducing inflammation, and improving vascular health, cognitive youth becomes sustainable rather than fragile. The chapters ahead will translate these metabolic principles into specific strategies for memory, focus, and long-term brain protection.

Ethan noticed something unexpected

Ethan had always relied on his mind. It was his sharpness, his ability to think quickly and solve problems, that defined his success. But somewhere in his early forties, that sharpness began to dull. Afternoons became a mental battle. Focus slipped. Simple decisions felt heavier than they should have.

At first, Ethan blamed workload. Then stress. Then age. Coffee became his crutch, sugar his comfort. Short bursts of clarity were followed by deeper crashes. He pushed harder, believing discipline alone would carry him through. It didn't.

One morning, after waking up already exhausted, Ethan realized something wasn't right. His mind felt starved, not tired. He began learning about how the brain uses energy—not motivation, not willpower, but fuel. The idea unsettled him. He had been feeding his body constantly, yet starving his brain of stability.

Small changes came first. Fewer spikes. More consistency. Better sleep. Movement that energized instead of drained him.

Slowly, the crashes softened. His mind stopped swinging between extremes. Focus returned—not explosively, but steadily. Weeks later, Ethan noticed something unexpected. He could think longer without fatigue. Conversations felt effortless again. He no longer needed constant stimulation to stay alert. His brain felt reliable, like a well-tuned engine instead of a temperamental machine.

The biggest shift wasn't physical—it was psychological. Ethan stopped blaming himself for fatigue. He understood that his brain had been doing the best it could with unstable fuel. Once the conditions changed, performance followed naturally.

Months passed, and his confidence returned—not the anxious kind driven by adrenaline, but the calm confidence of mental stability. He trusted his mind again. It showed up when needed, rested when allowed, and recovered quickly.

Ethan's transformation didn't come from pushing harder. It came from fueling smarter. His story reflects a truth many overlook: cognitive decline often begins as an energy problem, not a character flaw.

This chapter is an invitation to rethink how you power your mind. Your brain is not failing you—it is responding to the conditions you create. When energy becomes stable, clarity follows.

Mental sharpness is not reserved for the young or the lucky. It belongs to those who understand how to fuel it. And once that understanding takes hold, cognitive youth becomes not a hope, but a predictable outcome.

Chapter 4

Inflammation, Brain Aging & Neuroprotection

Inflammation is one of the most underestimated forces driving brain aging. While often associated with pain, injury, or illness, inflammation also operates quietly at a low grade for years, subtly altering brain structure and function long before symptoms appear. Neuroinflammation—chronic inflammation within the brain—disrupts neural communication, damages synapses, impairs energy metabolism, and accelerates cognitive decline. Understanding and controlling inflammation is therefore central to preserving cognitive youth.

The immune system plays a dual role in brain health. Acute inflammation is protective, helping eliminate pathogens and repair damaged tissue. However, when inflammation becomes chronic, it shifts from a healing mechanism to a destructive force. Persistent inflammatory signaling exposes neurons to cytokines and oxidative stress that interfere with neurotransmission and impair neuroplasticity. Over time, this inflammatory environment erodes cognitive resilience.

Microglia, the brain's resident immune cells, are central to neuroinflammation. In a healthy state, microglia monitor neural tissue and remove damaged cells. Under chronic stress, poor metabolic conditions, or repeated inflammatory exposure, microglia become overactivated. This hyperactivation leads to excessive synaptic pruning and neuronal damage, weakening neural networks essential for memory and focus.

Systemic inflammation often originates outside the brain but eventually crosses into the central nervous system. Poor diet, insulin resistance, gut permeability, chronic stress, sleep deprivation, and environmental toxins all contribute to a pro-inflammatory state. When the blood-brain barrier becomes compromised, inflammatory molecules enter the brain more easily, amplifying neuroinflammation and accelerating cognitive aging.

Oxidative stress is closely linked to inflammation. Reactive oxygen species are natural byproducts of metabolism, but when their production exceeds the brain's antioxidant defenses, they damage cellular membranes, mitochondria, and DNA. Neurons are particularly vulnerable due to their high metabolic demand and limited regenerative capacity. Chronic oxidative stress compounds inflammatory damage, creating a cycle that accelerates brain aging.

Inflammation directly impairs neurotransmitter balance. Pro-inflammatory cytokines reduce the synthesis of serotonin and dopamine while increasing excitotoxic signaling through glutamate. This imbalance contributes not only to cognitive decline but also to mood disorders, anxiety, and emotional instability. Cognitive youth depends on maintaining both structural integrity and neurochemical balance.

Metabolic health strongly influences inflammatory load. Insulin resistance, visceral fat accumulation, and blood sugar volatility all promote inflammatory signaling. Adipose tissue itself acts as an inflammatory organ, releasing cytokines that affect the brain. Improving metabolic function reduces systemic inflammation and restores a more protective neural environment.

Sleep plays a critical role in inflammation control. During deep sleep, inflammatory markers decrease and the brain clears metabolic waste through the glymphatic system. Chronic sleep disruption elevates inflammatory cytokines, weakens the blood-brain barrier, and increases vulnerability to neurodegeneration. Protecting sleep quality is therefore one of the most powerful anti-inflammatory interventions for brain longevity.

Stress is another potent inflammatory driver. Chronic

psychological stress elevates cortisol and sympathetic nervous system activity, both of which increase inflammatory signaling over time. Stress-related inflammation damages hippocampal neurons and accelerates cognitive decline. Nervous system regulation is essential for maintaining an anti-inflammatory brain environment.

Neuroprotection involves both reducing inflammatory inputs and enhancing the brain's resilience to unavoidable stressors. Antioxidant capacity, mitochondrial efficiency, vascular health, and neurotrophic signaling all contribute to neural defense. When these systems are supported, the brain can withstand transient inflammatory challenges without long-term damage.

This chapter establishes inflammation as a central modifiable factor in brain aging. Cognitive decline is not merely the result of time—it is often the result of prolonged inflammatory exposure. By reducing inflammation and strengthening neuroprotective systems, cognitive youth becomes sustainable across decades.

Her memory improved

When Olivia began forgetting words mid-sentence, she told herself it was stress. Life had been heavy for years—work deadlines, family obligations, sleepless nights. She had learned to function through exhaustion, mistaking survival for resilience. But something felt different now. Her mind felt noisy, scattered, and emotionally fragile.

She noticed her patience thinning. Small frustrations felt overwhelming. Even joyful moments seemed muted. Olivia wasn't depressed, but she wasn't herself either. Her thoughts felt inflamed—reactive, sharp, easily derailed. She wondered when calm had become so difficult.

A routine medical visit introduced a concept she had never considered: chronic inflammation. Not infection. Not illness. Just persistent internal stress. As she began learning, pieces fell into place. Years of poor sleep, rushed meals, constant tension, and emotional overload had shaped her internal chemistry.

Olivia didn't change everything at once. She started with rest. Real rest. Then nourishment that felt grounding instead of stimulating. Gentle movement instead of punishment. Moments of quiet she once considered unproductive. Slowly, the noise in her mind softened.

Weeks later, she noticed she could pause again. React less. Think more clearly before responding. Her memory improved, but more importantly, her emotional steadiness returned. The sharp edges that once defined her days smoothed into clarity.

She realized that her brain had been under constant attack—not from failure, but from inflammation. Once the attack eased, her natural intelligence resurfaced. She hadn't lost herself. She had been protecting herself the only way she knew how.

Months later, Olivia felt mentally younger than she had in years. Not because life was easier, but because her brain was no longer fighting itself. Calm became accessible again. Focus returned. Creativity followed.

Her story is not about perfection. It is about relief. Relief that decline is not inevitable. Relief that clarity can return. Relief that the brain, when protected, remembers how to function well.

This chapter is a reminder that cognitive youth requires safety. A brain under constant threat cannot thrive. But when inflammation subsides, the brain does what it was designed to do—adapt, connect, and remain alive with possibility.

Your mind is not broken. It may simply be inflamed. And inflammation, unlike time, can be changed.

Chapter 5

Memory Systems: Protecting Learning, Recall & Cognitive Continuity

Memory is not a single function but a coordinated system involving multiple brain regions, biochemical pathways, and neural networks. It encompasses encoding, storage, consolidation, and retrieval—each stage dependent on metabolic stability, synaptic integrity, sleep architecture, and neurochemical balance. Cognitive youth depends heavily on preserving the efficiency of these processes. Memory decline is often interpreted as unavoidable aging, yet it is frequently the result of modifiable biological stressors that impair neural communication over time.

The hippocampus plays a central role in memory formation, particularly in converting short-term experiences into long-term storage. This region is highly sensitive to inflammation, stress hormones, metabolic disruption, and sleep deprivation. Chronic exposure to elevated cortisol damages hippocampal neurons, reducing their ability to encode new information. Over time, this leads to the common experience of remembering distant events clearly while struggling with recent recall. Protecting hippocampal integrity is therefore foundational to cognitive longevity. Memory encoding depends on attention. Information must first be processed deeply enough to form stable neural representations. Modern environments characterized by constant distraction, multitasking, and fragmented attention weaken encoding pathways. When attention is shallow or divided, memory traces remain weak and prone to loss. Cognitive youth requires deliberate engagement that allows information to be processed fully before being stored.

Synaptic plasticity underlies learning. When neurons fire together repeatedly, their connections strengthen through long-term potentiation, the primary biological mechanism of memory consolidation. This process depends on adequate energy supply, neurotransmitter balance, and structural integrity of synapses. Metabolic dysfunction, inflammation, and oxidative stress all interfere with synaptic signaling, impairing learning capacity even before noticeable memory loss appears.

Sleep is essential for memory consolidation. During slow-wave and REM sleep stages, recently encoded information is transferred from temporary storage in the hippocampus to distributed cortical networks for long-term retention. Sleep deprivation disrupts this transfer, leaving memories fragile and incomplete. Chronic sleep disruption therefore reduces both memory stability and learning efficiency. Consistent, high-quality sleep is one of the most powerful interventions for preserving cognitive function.

Neurotransmitters play distinct roles in memory processes. Acetylcholine supports attention and encoding, glutamate drives synaptic plasticity, dopamine reinforces learning through reward signaling, and GABA regulates neural noise to allow clear signal transmission. Imbalances in these systems—often driven by stress, poor nutrition, or metabolic dysfunction—impair memory formation and recall accuracy. Maintaining neurochemical stability is essential for cognitive longevity.

Aging also affects retrieval efficiency. Even when memories remain stored, access pathways can weaken if neural networks are underused. Retrieval itself strengthens memory circuits; recalling information reinforces the synaptic patterns that encode it. Conversely, lack of recall practice allows these pathways to degrade. Active engagement with learned material preserves accessibility across time.

Emotional state influences memory profoundly. Moderate emotional arousal enhances encoding through amygdala–hippocampal interaction, but chronic anxiety or stress disrupts consolidation and retrieval. Persistent stress hormones interfere with hippocampal signaling and bias memory toward threat-related content. Emotional regulation therefore supports both memory accuracy and cognitive stability.

Physical movement enhances memory by increasing cerebral blood flow, oxygen delivery, and neurotrophic factor release. Exercise stimulates hippocampal neurogenesis—the formation of new neurons—supporting learning and recall capacity. Sedentary behavior reduces this stimulation, accelerating memory decline. Movement acts as both a metabolic and structural intervention for brain longevity.

Nutrition supports memory through its effects on neurotransmitter synthesis, mitochondrial function, and inflammation control. Essential fatty acids maintain neuronal membrane fluidity, amino acids provide neurotransmitter precursors, and micronutrients support enzymatic processes underlying neural signaling. Deficiencies in these substrates impair memory efficiency long before structural decline becomes apparent.

Cognitive challenge preserves memory systems by maintaining network complexity. Learning new material, recalling information, and integrating knowledge stimulate synaptic growth and prevent pruning of underused pathways. Passive information consumption without retrieval or application produces minimal neural reinforcement. Memory is strengthened through use, not exposure.

This chapter establishes memory as an active biological process requiring continual reinforcement and support. Decline is not inevitable; it is often the result of disrupted encoding, consolidation, or retrieval pathways. By stabilizing these systems, cognitive continuity—the ability to retain and access knowledge across time—can be preserved well into advanced age.

He began learning new things

Thomas had always been the storyteller in his family. He remembered birthdays, details, shared jokes, and moments others forgot. His memory was his pride—a quiet proof of presence. But in his late sixties, something shifted. Names slipped. Dates blurred. Stories paused mid-sentence as if someone had dimmed the lights inside his mind.

At first, he laughed it off. Everyone forgets. Everyone ages. But privately, he felt fear. Not of illness, but of disappearance. If memory faded, what remained of who he had been? He began withdrawing slightly, avoiding situations where recall might fail. Silence felt safer than uncertainty.

One afternoon, his granddaughter asked him to tell her about his childhood. As he began, memories returned—not all at once, but in fragments. Smells, sounds, scenes. She listened intently, asking questions that pulled details forward. For the first time in months, Thomas felt his past reassemble itself.

That moment changed him. He realized memory was not simply stored—it was awakened. When he engaged with it, it strengthened. When ignored, it faded. He began revisiting old stories, writing fragments down, recalling names deliberately, practicing retrieval instead of fearing failure.

Weeks passed, and his confidence returned. Not perfection, but access. He noticed that memories surfaced more easily when he expected them to. Fear had been blocking recall as much as age. By trusting his mind again, he reopened pathways he thought were lost.

Thomas also began learning new things—simple at first. A language app. A musical rhythm. Each small success reinforced belief: his brain still worked. It still adapted. It still remembered how to remember.

Months later, Thomas stood at a family gathering telling a story from decades earlier. His voice carried warmth and clarity. As laughter followed, he felt something profound—not relief, but continuity. He was still himself. His memories were still reachable. Thomas's journey reveals a quiet truth. Memory is not erased overnight. It weakens when unused, when feared, when disconnected. But when invited back through attention and practice, it often returns.

This chapter is an invitation to reconnect with your own continuity. Your memories are not fragile artifacts—they are living networks that respond to engagement. When you revisit them, they strengthen. When you build new ones, they expand.

Cognitive youth is not only about future clarity. It is also about preserving the bridge between who you have been and who you continue to become. Memory is that bridge. And with care, it can endure.

Chapter 6

Attention & Focus: Preserving Mental Clarity in an Overstimulated World

Attention is the gateway to cognition. Every thought, memory, decision, and action depends first on the brain's ability to select and sustain focus. Without stable attention, learning weakens, memory encoding fails, emotional regulation deteriorates, and cognitive performance fragments. In the context of longevity, preserving attention is not merely about productivity—it is about maintaining the coherence and clarity of the mind itself. Cognitive youth depends heavily on the brain's capacity to sustain directed awareness despite internal and external distraction.

Attention operates through coordinated networks distributed across the prefrontal cortex, parietal lobes, and subcortical structures. These networks regulate selective focus, sustained attention, and executive control. With aging, metabolic stress, inflammation, sleep disruption, and chronic overstimulation weaken these circuits, reducing the brain's ability to filter irrelevant stimuli and maintain mental engagement. The result is distractibility, mental fatigue, and reduced cognitive endurance. Modern environments place unprecedented strain on attention systems. Constant notifications, multitasking demands, rapid information switching, and dopamine-driven digital engagement train the brain toward fragmentation rather than depth. Each interruption forces attentional networks to disengage and reorient, consuming metabolic energy and weakening sustained focus capacity. Over time, the brain adapts to shallow engagement, making prolonged concentration increasingly difficult.

Neurochemistry plays a central role in attention regulation. Dopamine supports motivation and goal-directed focus, norepinephrine enhances alertness, and acetylcholine stabilizes sustained attention. Imbalances in these neurotransmitters—often driven by sleep deprivation, stress, metabolic instability, or overstimulation—disrupt attentional control. Excessive dopamine stimulation from constant novelty-seeking behavior can paradoxically reduce baseline focus by desensitizing reward pathways.

Energy metabolism strongly influences attention. Sustained focus requires stable glucose delivery, efficient mitochondrial function, and adequate oxygenation. Blood sugar volatility, insulin resistance, and poor cerebral blood flow reduce neuronal efficiency, producing mental fatigue and attentional lapses. Cognitive endurance is therefore a metabolic phenomenon as much as a psychological one. Sleep quality determines attentional resilience. During restorative sleep, attentional networks recover metabolic resources and clear accumulated neural waste. Chronic sleep deprivation impairs prefrontal cortex function, reducing executive control and increasing susceptibility to distraction. Individuals often interpret this as lack of discipline, when it is frequently a biological limitation imposed by insufficient neural recovery.

Stress exerts a dual influence on attention. Acute stress can temporarily sharpen focus through increased catecholamine release, but chronic stress overwhelms attentional circuits and impairs executive regulation. Elevated cortisol disrupts prefrontal cortex signaling, shifting the brain toward reactive, survival-oriented processing. Sustained attention becomes difficult when the nervous system remains in a threat-responsive state.

Training attention restores neural efficiency. Practices that require sustained engagement—deep reading, focused problem-solving, skill acquisition, and mindfulness-based attention training—strengthen prefrontal networks and improve resistance to distraction. Like memory, attention follows the principle of use-dependent plasticity. What is practiced becomes easier; what is neglected deteriorates.

Movement enhances attentional capacity by increasing cerebral perfusion and neurotransmitter availability.

Rhythmic physical activity, particularly aerobic movement, supports dopamine and norepinephrine balance, improving sustained focus. Sedentary behavior reduces these benefits, contributing to attentional decline over time.

Emotional regulation also influences focus. Anxiety, rumination, and intrusive thoughts consume attentional bandwidth, leaving fewer resources available for cognitive tasks. Chronic emotional activation fragments attention and accelerates mental fatigue. Nervous system regulation therefore preserves both emotional stability and cognitive clarity.

Attention is not infinite; it is renewable. Periods of deep focus require subsequent recovery to restore neural resources. Continuous stimulation without rest exhausts attentional systems, leading to burnout-like cognitive states. Alternating focus with restoration supports long-term cognitive endurance and protects attentional networks from decline.

This chapter establishes attention as a central pillar of brain longevity. Cognitive youth depends not only on memory and energy but on the brain's ability to direct awareness intentionally. By protecting attentional systems from overstimulation, metabolic instability, and chronic stress, mental clarity can be preserved across the lifespan.

Lena now protects her attention

Lena used to lose hours inside her work. Ideas flowed, problems unraveled, and time seemed irrelevant. Focus had once felt natural, almost effortless. But somewhere in her late thirties, that ease disappeared. Her days became fractured—emails, alerts, messages, unfinished thoughts scattered across screens.

She noticed she could no longer stay with a single task. Even reading felt restless. Her mind jumped ahead, drifted away, returned tired. She blamed workload, then motivation, then herself. "I just can't concentrate like I used to," she admitted quietly.

One evening, after abandoning yet another project halfway through, Lena realized something deeper had changed. Her mind wasn't weak—it was overstimulated. Years of constant input had trained her brain to expect interruption. Silence felt unfamiliar. Stillness uncomfortable.

She decided to experiment. One task, no switching. Ten minutes. The first attempts felt unbearable. Her mind reached for distraction automatically. But she stayed. Breath steady, attention anchored. Ten minutes became fifteen. Then twenty.

Over weeks, something subtle shifted. Thoughts slowed. Depth returned. She could follow ideas again without losing them. The scattered noise that once filled her mind softened into clarity. Focus felt less forced, more available.

Lena also noticed emotional changes. Without constant interruption, she felt calmer. Less reactive. More present in conversations. She began finishing what she started, rediscovering satisfaction in completion. Confidence returned—not through achievement, but through continuity of attention.

Months later, Lena spent an afternoon immersed in creative work. When she looked up, hours had passed. The state she thought lost had returned—not identically, but mature, steadier. She realized focus had never disappeared; it had been retrained away.

Her journey revealed a truth rarely taught: attention is shaped by environment. When the brain lives in interruption, it becomes fragmented. When it lives in depth, it regains coherence. Focus is not personality—it is conditioning.

Lena now protects her attention the way others protect time or money. She understands it as the foundation of thought itself. With it, her mind feels whole. Without it, scattered.

This chapter is a reminder that mental clarity is recoverable. Even in overstimulated environments, attention can be rebuilt through deliberate practice. The brain remembers how to focus when given the chance.

Your attention is your presence. Where it rests shapes who you become. And when it is strengthened, cognitive youth becomes not just preserved—but experienced daily.

Chapter 7

Emotional Regulation: Mood, Stress & Cognitive Stability Across Time

Emotional regulation is a central yet often overlooked determinant of brain longevity. While cognition is frequently discussed in terms of memory, focus, or learning, the emotional environment in which the brain operates profoundly influences all cognitive processes. Chronic anxiety, persistent stress, mood instability, and emotional reactivity alter neural signaling, disrupt neurotransmitter balance, impair attention, and accelerate structural brain aging. Preserving cognitive youth therefore requires stabilizing emotional circuitry alongside intellectual function.

Emotion and cognition are biologically inseparable. The limbic system, particularly the amygdala and hippocampus, interacts continuously with the prefrontal cortex, the region responsible for executive control and rational processing. When emotional centers become overactivated, prefrontal regulation weakens, reducing decision-making clarity and cognitive flexibility. Chronic emotional dysregulation effectively shifts the brain from reflective processing toward reactive survival mode, limiting higher cognitive performance. Stress hormones are primary mediators of this shift. Cortisol and adrenaline are adaptive during acute challenges, enhancing vigilance and rapid response. However, prolonged elevation of these hormones damages neural tissue, particularly in the hippocampus and prefrontal cortex. Sustained cortisol exposure reduces synaptic density, impairs neurogenesis, and weakens memory encoding. Emotional stress thus directly accelerates cognitive aging through hormonal pathways.

Neurotransmitter balance also depends heavily on emotional state. Serotonin stabilizes mood and supports emotional resilience, dopamine reinforces motivation and reward processing, and GABA dampens excessive neural excitation. Chronic stress, sleep deprivation, inflammation, and metabolic dysfunction disrupt these systems, leading to anxiety, irritability, and mood volatility. Such instability consumes cognitive resources that would otherwise support attention and memory.

The nervous system operates along a continuum between sympathetic activation and parasympathetic restoration. Persistent sympathetic dominance, characterized by vigilance and tension, keeps the brain in threat-detection mode. In this state, attentional bias shifts toward perceived danger, reducing capacity for learning, creativity, and reflective thinking. Parasympathetic balance restores neural safety, allowing higher cognitive networks to function efficiently. Emotional regulation therefore depends on autonomic balance.

Emotional patterns are reinforced through neural plasticity. Repeated emotional responses strengthen corresponding neural circuits, making reactions more automatic over time. Chronic worry, rumination, or anger thus becomes neurologically ingrained. Conversely, practices that cultivate calm, perspective, and resilience reinforce stabilizing circuits. Emotional regulation is trainable because neural pathways adapt to repeated experience.

Sleep interacts strongly with emotional stability. During REM sleep, the brain processes emotional experiences and recalibrates limbic activity. Sleep deprivation heightens amygdala reactivity while reducing prefrontal control, increasing emotional volatility. Individuals often interpret this as mood disorder when it is partially a consequence of neural fatigue. Protecting sleep restores emotional equilibrium and cognitive clarity simultaneously.

Inflammation also affects mood regulation. Pro-inflammatory cytokines alter neurotransmitter metabolism and increase neural excitability, contributing to anxiety and depressive symptoms. Chronic inflammation therefore disrupts both emotional stability and cognitive function. Anti-inflammatory physiology supports psychological resilience as well as brain longevity.

Social connection is a powerful regulator of emotional circuitry. Cooperative interaction, trust, and supportive relationships activate neural pathways associated with safety and reward. Isolation increases stress hormones and inflammatory signaling, impairing emotional and cognitive health. Humans are neurologically designed for social regulation; connection stabilizes both mood and cognition.

Movement supports emotional regulation through multiple pathways. Physical activity modulates neurotransmitters, reduces cortisol, enhances blood flow, and increases neurotrophic factors. Regular movement is associated with improved mood stability and reduced anxiety, demonstrating the interdependence of physical and emotional brain health.

Cognitive reframing and mindfulness-based awareness strengthen prefrontal regulation over limbic reactivity. Observing emotional states without immediate reaction increases neural flexibility and reduces automatic stress responses. Over time, this practice reshapes emotional circuits, enhancing stability and cognitive resilience.

Emotional regulation does not eliminate feeling; it stabilizes response. A brain capable of experiencing emotion without chronic dysregulation preserves neural resources for cognition, creativity, and learning. When emotional circuitry is balanced, cognitive networks operate without interference, sustaining clarity across time.

This chapter establishes emotional regulation as a cornerstone of cognitive longevity. The aging brain is shaped not only by metabolism and memory but by emotional climate. Stabilizing mood, reducing chronic stress, and reinforcing resilience preserve both neural structure and cognitive function across decades.

Slowing breath during agitation

Marcus had always believed he was rational. He prided himself on logic, decisions, and composure. But beneath that surface lived constant tension. Deadlines, expectations, responsibilities—all carried silently. He rarely named it stress; he called it drive.

Over years, that drive hardened into restlessness. Sleep became shallow. Patience thinned. Small frustrations sparked disproportionate reactions. His mind felt crowded, thoughts looping, emotions close to the surface. He noticed memory slips and scattered focus, which he blamed on workload. But deep down, he sensed something else—instability. One evening, after reacting sharply to someone he cared about, Marcus felt a quiet realization: his mind was not calm. It had not been calm for years. He had normalized tension so completely he no longer recognized it as abnormal.

He began exploring how emotion shapes cognition. The idea unsettled him. He had thought intellect stood apart from feeling. Yet he saw clearly: constant stress had been draining clarity, fragmenting attention, exhausting memory. His brain had been operating in threat mode, not thought mode.

Marcus began small experiments. Slowing breath during agitation. Pausing before response. Allowing silence instead of filling it. At first, these moments felt unfamiliar, even uncomfortable. But they introduced something he had not felt in years—space.

Weeks later, he noticed his reactions softening. Irritation passed more quickly. Thoughts felt less crowded. Conversations required less effort. The mind he had once relied on began to feel accessible again, not forced.

He also rediscovered rest. Not collapse from exhaustion, but intentional recovery. Sleep deepened. Mornings felt clearer. Emotional swings leveled. The stability he had always sought through control emerged through regulation instead.

Months passed, and Marcus recognized a profound change. He was not less driven or capable. He was steadier. Decisions came with clarity rather than urgency. Memory sharpened. Focus extended. His mind felt organized instead of pressured.

He realized emotional calm was not weakness—it was infrastructure. Without it, cognition faltered. With it, intelligence flowed naturally. He had spent years strengthening thought while neglecting the emotional system that sustained it.

Marcus's story reflects a hidden truth: many people attribute cognitive decline to age or workload when it arises from emotional overload. When the nervous system stabilizes, clarity returns. The brain remembers how to think well once it no longer defends constantly.

This chapter is an invitation to treat emotional stability as cognitive training. Calm is not absence of emotion; it is balanced emotion. And balance preserves neural resources needed for memory, attention, and reasoning.

Your mind does not separate thought from feeling. They share the same networks. When emotion stabilizes, cognition strengthens. And in that stability, cognitive youth endures.

Chapter 8

Social Connection & Purpose: The Brain's Need for Meaningful Engagement

Human cognition evolved within social environments. The brain developed not only to process information but to interpret relationships, coordinate behavior, and navigate complex social networks. As a result, social connection and sense of purpose are not psychological luxuries; they are biological requirements for optimal brain function. Longevity research consistently shows that individuals with strong social bonds and meaningful roles maintain cognitive health longer than those who experience isolation or purposelessness. Brain longevity therefore depends not only on metabolic and neurological factors but on relational and motivational engagement across the lifespan.

Social interaction stimulates multiple cognitive domains simultaneously. Language processing, memory recall, emotional interpretation, attention shifting, and executive planning all activate during meaningful conversation or cooperative activity. This multidimensional stimulation strengthens neural connectivity across distributed brain networks. Isolation, by contrast, deprives the brain of this integrated activation, allowing synaptic pathways associated with social cognition and emotional regulation to weaken over time. Reduced social engagement thus accelerates cognitive decline through disuse.

The prefrontal cortex and limbic system are particularly responsive to social experience. Trust, cooperation, and shared attention activate reward pathways involving dopamine and oxytocin, reinforcing neural circuits associated with safety and motivation. Chronic loneliness elevates stress hormones, increases inflammatory signaling, and alters neurotransmitter balance. The brain interprets social isolation as a threat state, shifting neural resources toward vigilance rather than cognitive growth. Sustained loneliness therefore becomes biologically toxic to cognitive longevity.

Purpose further amplifies cognitive resilience. A sense of direction or contribution organizes neural activity around meaningful goals, sustaining motivation and attentional engagement. Purpose-driven behavior recruits executive networks in the prefrontal cortex, enhancing planning, memory integration, and emotional regulation. Individuals with clear roles or goals maintain higher cognitive performance because their brains remain engaged in adaptive problem-solving and decision-making processes.

Motivation itself is neurologically protective. Dopaminergic pathways associated with anticipation and reward reinforce learning and neuroplasticity. Purposeful activity repeatedly activates these pathways, preserving synaptic strength and neural responsiveness. Conversely, absence of meaningful engagement reduces dopaminergic activity, contributing to apathy, reduced curiosity, and cognitive stagnation. The brain remains youthful when it anticipates relevance and contribution.

Social cognition also supports emotional regulation. Interpersonal feedback helps calibrate emotional responses, reducing rumination and anxiety. Supportive relationships buffer stress responses, lowering cortisol and inflammatory markers. Through shared experience, the brain receives signals of safety that stabilize neural networks governing mood and attention. Emotional stability gained through connection indirectly protects cognitive systems.

Communication demands memory and linguistic precision. Recalling shared experiences, names, and contextual details during interaction exercises hippocampal and cortical memory circuits. Frequent social engagement therefore functions as natural memory training. In contrast, reduced interaction decreases retrieval practice, allowing access pathways to weaken. Cognitive decline observed in isolation often reflects loss of use rather than loss of capacity.

Purpose and connection also influence behavior patterns that support brain health. Individuals engaged in meaningful roles are more likely to maintain routines, physical activity, and cognitive challenge. Motivation derived from contribution reinforces health-supportive behaviors that protect neural integrity. Thus, purpose operates both directly through neural activation and indirectly through lifestyle regulation.

Aging often introduces transitions—retirement, relocation, bereavement—that disrupt established roles and social networks. Without intentional replacement of engagement, cognitive stimulation declines. Brain longevity therefore requires proactive cultivation of connection and meaning across life stages. Social and purposeful engagement must evolve rather than diminish with age.

Neuroplasticity remains responsive to relational experience throughout life. New relationships, collaborative learning, mentoring, volunteering, and shared creative activities stimulate network growth even in later decades. The social brain retains adaptability, provided it remains engaged. Longevity does not reduce the need for connection; it increases its importance. Cognitive identity is partly constructed through interaction. The self is reinforced by recognition, dialogue, and shared narrative. Social withdrawal reduces these reinforcing signals, contributing to perceived cognitive decline. Engagement sustains not only function but identity continuity. The brain remains oriented and active when it participates in relational environments.

This chapter establishes social connection and purpose as structural supports for cognitive longevity. The brain thrives when embedded in meaningful networks of interaction and contribution. Isolation and purposelessness, by contrast, accelerate neural decline through reduced stimulation and increased stress. Sustained engagement preserves cognitive vitality across the lifespan.

He felt present again

After retirement, Harold expected relief. Decades of responsibility had ended. Schedules loosened. Obligations faded. For a while, the quiet felt deserved. But months passed, and the silence deepened. Days blurred without structure. Conversations grew infrequent. The world seemed to move without needing him.

Harold noticed changes he couldn't name at first. Memory slips. Slower thinking. A sense of dullness where alertness once lived. He assumed age was finally claiming its due. Without work, he reasoned, the mind naturally slowed.

One afternoon, a former colleague called asking for advice. The request surprised him. As Harold explained, something awakened—clarity, confidence, engagement. His thoughts organized quickly. Memories surfaced effortlessly. For an hour, he felt exactly as he had years before.

After the call, the realization lingered: his mind had not faded. It had rested too long without use. What he missed was not activity alone, but relevance. He had lost the feeling of being needed.

Harold began small. Offering help to neighbors. Joining community meetings. Sharing skills he had once taken for granted. Each interaction reignited mental pathways. Conversations demanded recall, planning, attention. His days regained rhythm. His thoughts regained sharpness.

Weeks later, he noticed the fog lifting. Memory improved. Focus steadied. More importantly, he felt present again—anchored in relationships and contribution. The quiet isolation that had seemed restful now appeared draining. Engagement restored energy.

Harold also discovered joy in mentoring younger individuals entering his former field. Explaining concepts required organization of knowledge. Questions challenged him. Learning returned—not formal, but alive. His brain responded as if reactivated.

Months passed, and Harold recognized a profound shift. He no longer saw retirement as decline. It had been disconnection. Once connection returned, cognition followed. He had mistaken absence of role for loss of capacity.

His story reveals a subtle truth: the brain is relational. It sharpens when shared. It dulls when unused in isolation. Meaning and connection act as cognitive nutrients. Without them, even healthy brains slow.

Harold's mind had not aged suddenly. It had quieted from lack of engagement. Once invited back into participation, it responded immediately. Clarity was not lost; it was dormant.

This chapter is an invitation to recognize the brain's need for relevance. Purpose is not an abstract idea—it is neural activation. Connection is not social luxury—it is cognitive exercise. The mind remains vibrant when it matters to others and itself.

Your cognitive future is shaped not only by what you think, but by who you think with and for. Engagement sustains identity, memory, and clarity. And when purpose endures, cognitive youth follows naturally.

Chapter 9

Lifestyle Architecture: Daily Habits That Preserve Cognitive Youth

Cognitive longevity is not sustained by isolated interventions but by consistent patterns embedded in daily life. The brain responds continuously to lifestyle inputs—sleep timing, nutrition quality, movement patterns, cognitive engagement, stress exposure, and environmental stimulation. These recurring conditions shape neural physiology over years and decades, determining whether cognitive function stabilizes or declines. Lifestyle architecture refers to the intentional design of daily behaviors that support long-term brain health. When aligned with neural biology, these habits create cumulative protection for memory, attention, emotional stability, and mental clarity.

Habitual behaviors influence brain structure through repetition. Neural circuits activated regularly strengthen, while unused pathways weaken. This principle of use-dependent plasticity means that daily routines exert powerful effects on cognitive resilience. Consistent intellectual engagement reinforces prefrontal and hippocampal networks, whereas passive or repetitive routines reduce neural complexity. Cognitive youth therefore depends on embedding stimulation and novelty within ordinary life rather than relying solely on occasional training.

Sleep timing anchors lifestyle architecture. Circadian rhythms regulate hormone release, neurotransmitter balance, and metabolic efficiency within the brain. Irregular sleep schedules disrupt these rhythms, impairing memory consolidation, emotional regulation, and attention stability. Consistent sleep–wake timing strengthens circadian alignment, allowing neural repair and metabolic clearance processes to operate predictably. Over years, this stability protects cognitive systems from cumulative disruption.

Nutritional patterns shape brain metabolism daily. Regular intake of nutrient-dense foods supports neurotransmitter synthesis, mitochondrial function, and inflammation control. Conversely, frequent consumption of ultra-processed foods, excessive sugars, or erratic meal timing destabilizes energy supply and promotes inflammatory signaling. The brain requires metabolic consistency more than caloric excess. Habitual nutrition patterns therefore influence cognitive performance across time.

Movement patterns also determine neural vitality. Regular physical activity enhances cerebral blood flow, oxygenation, and neurotrophic factor production, supporting synaptic growth and neurogenesis. Sedentary habits reduce these benefits, accelerating structural and metabolic decline. Importantly, daily movement need not be extreme; consistent moderate activity produces cumulative neural protection. Lifestyle architecture integrates movement as a normal part of routine rather than an occasional effort.

Cognitive engagement embedded in routine maintains neural complexity. Activities requiring planning, problem-solving, learning, or creative expression stimulate distributed brain networks. Passive consumption without interaction produces minimal reinforcement. When daily life includes thinking challenges, conversation, learning, and skill practice, cognitive systems remain active and adaptive. The brain thrives when stimulation is continuous rather than sporadic.

Stress exposure patterns shape neural aging. Chronic unpredictability, overload, or emotional strain elevate cortisol and inflammatory markers, damaging hippocampal and prefrontal structures. Daily habits that include recovery—rest, reflection, calm exposure to nature, or restorative practices—counterbalance stress physiology. Over years, this balance determines whether emotional and cognitive circuits remain stable or degrade under pressure. Environmental stimulation influences neural activation. Sensory variety, natural light exposure, spatial navigation, and novelty enrich cognitive processing. Monotonous or confined environments reduce sensory input, diminishing neural engagement. Lifestyle architecture considers physical surroundings as cognitive inputs, encouraging variation and exploration that stimulate spatial and perceptual networks.

Social interaction incorporated into routine reinforces relational cognition and emotional regulation. Frequent meaningful conversation, shared tasks, or collaborative activities stimulate memory, language, and executive networks. Isolation reduces this activation, accelerating decline. Consistent relational engagement therefore becomes a daily cognitive habit rather than an occasional event.

Attention management also depends on habitual structure. Environments filled with constant interruption fragment focus, weakening attentional endurance. Routines that include uninterrupted work periods, device-free time, and single-task engagement preserve prefrontal regulation. Over time, attentional stability becomes conditioned by these patterns. Lifestyle architecture protects focus by controlling exposure to distraction.

Identity reinforcement occurs through repeated behavior. Individuals who routinely engage in learning, movement, connection, and reflection strengthen self-perception as cognitively capable. This identity influences motivation and behavior continuity. When lifestyle habits align with cognitive preservation, the brain experiences consistency between intention and action, reinforcing neural stability.

Longevity emerges from accumulation. Each day's inputs may appear minor, but their repetition shapes neural physiology across decades. Lifestyle architecture recognizes that cognitive youth is built gradually through sustained alignment between behavior and biology. By embedding brain-supportive habits into daily life, individuals create conditions in which cognition remains resilient without constant effort.

This chapter establishes daily lifestyle patterns as the operational layer of brain longevity. While neuroplasticity, metabolism, inflammation, and emotion provide mechanisms, lifestyle determines exposure. Cognitive youth persists when everyday habits consistently reinforce neural health rather than undermine it.

Her thoughts organized naturally

Eleanor had always believed big changes required big effort. Health meant strict plans, sudden transformations, bursts of motivation. But in her early sixties, she noticed her mind growing inconsistent. Some days clear, others foggy. She searched for dramatic solutions—supplements, programs, intense regimens—but nothing lasted.

One morning, she realized her days lacked rhythm. Sleep shifted nightly. Meals were rushed or skipped. Movement happened irregularly. Conversations had dwindled. Her life contained no stable patterns. Her mind reflected that instability—sometimes sharp, sometimes dull, never predictable.

Instead of pursuing another overhaul, Eleanor began with structure. Waking at the same time. Eating regularly. Walking daily. Reading each evening. Calling a friend weekly. These changes felt almost trivial. Yet weeks later, she sensed something different—steadiness.

Her mind no longer fluctuated wildly. Memory slips decreased. Focus returned gradually. She noticed she could sustain thought longer without fatigue. The chaos she once blamed on age had mirrored the chaos of her routine.

Encouraged, Eleanor added small cognitive challenges. Learning new recipes. Navigating unfamiliar routes. Practicing memory recall during conversation. None felt dramatic. But together, they reshaped her days. Life gained texture. The mind followed. Months passed, and Eleanor recognized a profound shift. She felt reliable to herself. Her thoughts organized naturally. Emotional swings softened. Cognitive clarity no longer depended on motivation; it emerged from consistency.

She realized she had misunderstood change. The brain did not require heroic effort—it required stable input. When daily life aligned with biology, cognition stabilized automatically. Her mind had been responding honestly to irregular conditions.

Eleanor also noticed identity changes. She began seeing herself as someone engaged, curious, capable. This self-image reinforced habits effortlessly. Structure no longer felt restrictive; it felt supportive. Her lifestyle became cognitive infrastructure.

Looking back, Eleanor saw that decline had not arrived suddenly. It had crept through inconsistency. Once patterns stabilized, clarity returned without force. She had not reclaimed youth, but continuity—a steady mind across days.

Her story illustrates a quiet truth: the brain reflects routine. Stability outside becomes stability inside. Lifestyle architecture is not discipline alone; it is alignment. When life becomes rhythmical, cognition becomes reliable.

This chapter is an invitation to redesign daily patterns gently but intentionally. Cognitive youth does not demand perfection.

It requires consistency. Small habits repeated across years shape neural destiny more than occasional extremes.

Your brain lives inside your days. Change the days, and the brain changes with them. And when patterns support biology, mental clarity becomes the natural state rather than the exception.

Chapter 10

Lifelong Brain Resilience: Protecting Cognitive Youth Across Decades

Cognitive longevity ultimately depends on resilience—the brain's capacity to withstand stress, adapt to change, and maintain function across time despite biological aging. While previous chapters have addressed individual drivers of brain health such as metabolism, inflammation, memory, attention, and lifestyle patterns, long-term protection emerges from integrating these elements into a durable neural environment. Brain resilience is not the absence of decline pressures; it is the presence of protective systems strong enough to counter them continuously.

Aging introduces cumulative biological challenges to the brain. Mitochondrial efficiency gradually decreases, oxidative stress accumulates, vascular elasticity declines, and neurochemical balance shifts. These changes are natural aspects of aging physiology. However, the rate at which they influence cognition varies dramatically depending on protective factors. Individuals with strong neural resilience often maintain cognitive function far beyond chronological expectations, demonstrating that aging trajectory is modifiable. Neural reserve represents one dimension of resilience. It refers to the structural capacity of the brain—synaptic density, neuronal connectivity, and network complexity—developed through lifelong cognitive engagement. Brains with greater reserve tolerate age-related changes without functional impairment because redundant pathways compensate for localized decline. Education, learning, novelty, and intellectual challenge across life contribute significantly to this reserve.

Cognitive reserve complements structural reserve by reflecting efficiency and adaptability of neural networks. Even when structural changes occur, flexible networks reorganize function through alternative pathways. Neuroplasticity underlies this adaptability. Continuous learning and cognitive stimulation maintain network flexibility, allowing the brain to reroute processing when primary circuits weaken. Resilient cognition therefore depends on sustained neural adaptability rather than static preservation.

Metabolic resilience also determines long-term brain protection. Stable glucose regulation, mitochondrial health, and vascular integrity ensure consistent energy availability across decades. Brains that maintain metabolic flexibility tolerate physiological aging better than those already compromised by insulin resistance or vascular impairment. Supporting metabolic health throughout life establishes a foundation for cognitive endurance in later years.

Inflammatory resilience further protects neural tissue. The ability to regulate immune responses and limit chronic inflammation preserves synaptic integrity and neurotransmitter balance. Individuals with lower systemic inflammatory burden show slower cognitive aging and reduced neurodegenerative risk. Anti-inflammatory physiology results from sustained lifestyle patterns rather than late intervention alone, emphasizing the importance of long-term alignment.

Stress resilience is equally critical. The brain's response to adversity shapes hormonal exposure and neural wear over time. Individuals capable of recovering quickly from stress maintain healthier prefrontal and hippocampal structures. Emotional regulation, supportive relationships, and restorative practices reinforce this resilience. Chronic unresolved stress, by contrast, accelerates structural brain aging regardless of other protective factors.

Sleep resilience supports neural maintenance across decades. Consistent restorative sleep enables metabolic waste clearance, synaptic repair, and memory consolidation nightly. Lifelong sleep disruption accumulates neural damage gradually, contributing to later cognitive decline. Protecting sleep quality throughout life therefore functions as continuous neuroprotection rather than episodic recovery. Behavioral adaptability represents another layer of resilience. The brain thrives when individuals adjust habits in response to changing physiology. Nutritional needs, activity levels, cognitive demands, and recovery requirements evolve with age. Adaptive behavior ensures alignment between lifestyle and biological state, preserving neural efficiency. Rigidity in habits despite physiological change accelerates mismatch and decline.

Purpose and engagement maintain motivational resilience. Individuals who remain mentally active, socially connected, and goal-oriented preserve cognitive drive that sustains neural activation. Motivation fuels engagement, and engagement reinforces neural networks. This positive cycle supports brain vitality even in advanced age. Disengagement breaks this cycle, reducing stimulation and accelerating decline.

Environmental resilience also influences brain aging. Exposure to enriched, varied environments stimulates sensory and cognitive networks. Monotony reduces stimulation, weakening neural activation. Lifelong exploration, novelty, and adaptive challenge reinforce neural complexity and resilience across decades.

Importantly, resilience accumulates gradually. Protective factors applied consistently across life build neural strength long before aging pressures intensify. Conversely, neglect of these factors reduces reserve, leaving the brain vulnerable when decline pressures increase. Cognitive longevity therefore reflects lifelong preparation rather than late correction.

The goal of brain longevity is not to prevent all change but to maintain function despite change. Resilient brains compensate, adapt, and reorganize. They preserve identity, memory, and clarity even as biological aging progresses. This capacity defines cognitive youth more than chronological age alone.

This final chapter establishes resilience as the integrating principle of cognitive longevity. By strengthening neural reserve, metabolic stability, inflammatory control, stress recovery, and adaptive engagement across life, the brain remains capable, flexible, and clear across decades. Lifelong cognitive youth is therefore not accidental—it is built.

Younger colleagues sought his perspective

Samuel had spent his life solving problems. Engineering projects, complex systems, intricate designs—his mind thrived on challenge. Even in his seventies, he remained intellectually active, reading, building, questioning. People often remarked on his sharpness, attributing it to natural intelligence.

But Samuel knew his mind had not always felt stable. In his fifties, after years of relentless work and poor sleep, he noticed lapses—misplaced details, slowed recall, scattered focus. The changes frightened him. His identity had always been tied to clarity. If that faded, who was he?

Instead of accepting decline, Samuel became curious. He studied how the brain ages and what protects it. The realization struck him deeply: cognition was not fixed. It was responsive. His brain reflected how he had lived, and it could reflect new conditions.

He began rebuilding slowly. Sleep became priority rather than afterthought. Movement replaced long sedentary stretches. Learning expanded beyond work into new domains. Social conversations deepened. Stress responses softened. None of these changes were dramatic alone, but together they reshaped his mind.

Years passed, and Samuel noticed something unexpected. While peers complained of mental decline, his clarity strengthened. He learned faster, reasoned deeply, remembered well. Aging did not erase capability—it revealed the strength he had built.

In his eighties, Samuel still approached problems with curiosity. Younger colleagues sought his perspective. He felt mentally present, not preserved but evolving. His mind adapted gracefully to slower pace without losing precision. Resilience had replaced fear.

Samuel understood that cognitive youth was not about remaining unchanged. It was about remaining functional despite change. His brain had aged biologically, yet remained capable because protective systems were strong. He had built reserve long before he needed it.

Looking back, Samuel saw clearly: his mind was not sharp by chance. It was shaped by decades of alignment between behavior and biology. Every habit, challenge, recovery, and connection had reinforced resilience. Aging revealed that foundation.

Samuel's story illustrates the essence of this book. Cognitive longevity is cumulative. It emerges from repeated investment in neural health across time. When resilience is built early and maintained consistently, the brain withstands aging pressures without losing identity.

His clarity in later years was not youth preserved—it was resilience expressed. He remained himself, thinking, remembering, creating. Aging changed his pace, not his presence.

This chapter closes with a simple truth: the brain you live with later is the brain you build now. Resilience grows from consistent care. And when built across years, cognitive youth endures naturally into age.

Chapter 11

Cognitive Renewal: Rebuilding the Brain at Any Age

The concept of cognitive decline has historically implied irreversibility, suggesting that once neural function deteriorates, restoration is limited or impossible. Contemporary neuroscience challenges this assumption. The adult brain retains the capacity for structural and functional renewal throughout life, provided that biological conditions support neuroplasticity, metabolic repair, and synaptic regeneration. Cognitive renewal refers to the deliberate activation of these restorative mechanisms to rebuild neural efficiency, even after periods of decline.

Neural networks are dynamic rather than fixed. Synapses form and dissolve in response to activity patterns, metabolic conditions, and environmental stimulation. When cognitive engagement increases, previously weakened circuits can strengthen again through long-term potentiation. This process does not require youth; it requires activation. Even in advanced age, repeated stimulation of neural pathways promotes synaptic reinforcement and functional recovery. Neurogenesis contributes to cognitive renewal. While once believed to cease after childhood, new neuron formation continues in the hippocampus across adulthood, particularly when stimulated by physical activity, enriched environments, and learning. These new neurons integrate into memory circuits, enhancing learning capacity and cognitive flexibility. Decline in neurogenesis often reflects environmental deprivation rather than chronological inevitability.

Metabolic repair supports neural rebuilding. Neurons depend on mitochondrial function and stable energy supply to maintain synaptic activity. When metabolic conditions improve—through stable glucose regulation, improved oxygen delivery, and reduced inflammation—neuronal efficiency increases. Cognitive improvement observed after metabolic intervention demonstrates the brain's capacity to recover function when energy deficits resolve.

Synaptic restoration also depends on reducing inhibitory pressures such as chronic inflammation and oxidative stress. Persistent inflammatory signaling suppresses neuroplasticity and damages neural membranes. Anti-inflammatory physiology allows synaptic repair processes to proceed, enabling network recovery. Removing barriers to plasticity is as important as providing stimulation for renewal.

Learning drives structural brain change across the lifespan. Acquisition of new skills increases gray matter density in relevant cortical regions and strengthens connectivity between distributed networks. Even late-life learning produces measurable neural expansion. The brain responds to demand; when challenged, it reorganizes to meet requirements. Cognitive stagnation reflects absence of challenge rather than absence of capacity.

Emotional state influences neural rebuilding. Chronic fear or hopelessness suppresses neuroplasticity through stress hormones that inhibit synaptic growth. Positive expectancy and engagement activate reward pathways that reinforce learning and adaptation. Psychological readiness therefore shapes biological renewal potential. Belief in possibility supports neural change.

Sleep facilitates neural repair essential for cognitive renewal. During deep sleep, synaptic homeostasis recalibrates neural strength, and metabolic waste is cleared. Adequate sleep restores conditions necessary for learning-induced plasticity. Chronic sleep deprivation prevents neural rebuilding by maintaining fatigue and inflammatory signaling. Restoration requires recovery cycles as much as stimulation.

Physical movement remains a powerful catalyst for neural regeneration. Aerobic activity increases brain-derived neurotrophic factor and cerebral blood flow, supporting synaptic growth and neuron survival. Movement-induced neurotrophic signaling enhances learning capacity and memory recovery. Cognitive renewal often accompanies physical activation because both share biological substrates.

Environmental enrichment stimulates broad neural activation. Exposure to varied sensory, cognitive, and social inputs increases synaptic complexity and network integration. Monotonous environments reduce stimulation, limiting plasticity. Renewal therefore requires varied engagement that challenges perception, cognition, and interaction simultaneously.

Importantly, cognitive renewal does not imply returning to a previous state but achieving functional improvement relative to current conditions. The brain adapts to present inputs rather than past baselines. Restoration thus means enhancing clarity, memory, and focus beyond decline levels, not recreating earlier neural states. Progress remains possible across all ages.

Motivation and persistence determine renewal success. Neural change requires repeated activation over time. Intermittent effort produces limited adaptation, whereas sustained engagement remodels networks durably. Cognitive renewal is therefore a process rather than an event, unfolding gradually through consistent stimulation and supportive physiology.

This chapter establishes cognitive renewal as a realistic and biologically grounded possibility. Decline does not eliminate plasticity; it often reflects underuse or adverse conditions. By restoring metabolic support, reducing inhibition, and increasing engagement, the brain rebuilds functional capacity across the lifespan. Cognitive youth can therefore re-emerge even after loss.

After his stroke, Victor believed his mind was gone. Words tangled. Memory fractured. Thoughts moved slowly, like objects through water. Doctors spoke carefully about recovery potential, but Victor heard only limitation. He had built his life on mental precision; now that precision seemed erased.

Victor began to understand renewal differently

The early weeks were filled with frustration. Simple tasks required effort that felt humiliating. He avoided conversation, ashamed of pauses and mistakes. Inside, he mourned the person he had been—articulate, sharp, confident. That identity felt unreachable.

Rehabilitation began gently. Naming objects. Repeating phrases. Remembering sequences. The exercises felt childish, far removed from his former complexity. Yet something unexpected occurred: improvement. Small, fragile, but real. Words surfaced more easily. Memory held longer.

Therapists explained the brain could rewire. Victor resisted the idea at first. How could damaged tissue rebuild? But daily practice revealed change. Pathways formed where none seemed possible. Effort produced adaptation. The mind responded to demand.

Months passed, and Victor expanded challenges. Reading again. Writing short notes. Holding conversations despite imperfections. Each success strengthened confidence. His brain felt less broken, more reorganizing. Loss remained, but function returned.

One afternoon, while explaining a story to his grandson, Victor realized he was speaking fluidly. Not perfectly, but naturally. The moment stunned him. His mind had not vanished—it had rerouted. Identity persisted through adaptation.

Victor began to understand renewal differently. He was not restoring the exact brain he had before. He was building a new one from surviving networks. That realization replaced grief with determination. Recovery became construction rather than repair.

Years later, Victor still spoke slowly, but thoughtfully. His memory differed, but worked. He solved problems with patience instead of speed. People often described him as wise rather than sharp. He recognized the distinction: his cognition had changed, not disappeared.

Victor's journey revealed that the brain does not surrender easily. Even after injury, it seeks new routes. When supported and challenged, it rebuilds function beyond expectation. Renewal may not restore the past, but it restores capability.

His story extends beyond injury. Many people experience quieter forms of cognitive loss—stress, fatigue, aging. Like Victor, they assume permanence. Yet the brain remains adaptable. Underuse and adversity conceal capacity that can re-emerge with activation.

Victor once believed his mind had ended. Instead, it transformed. He discovered that cognition is not fixed structure but living process. When engaged persistently, it reshapes itself to continue functioning.

This chapter closes with a powerful truth: cognitive renewal is possible at any age and after significant decline. The brain responds to stimulation, support, and persistence. Loss does not define its future. Engagement does.

Your mind is not static. Even now, it is capable of rebuilding. And when renewal begins, cognitive youth can reappear in new form—adapted, resilient, and alive.

Epilogue

Cognitive Youth as a Lifelong Practice

The preservation of cognitive youth is not achieved through a single intervention, stage of life, or period of effort. It is the cumulative outcome of sustained alignment between biology, behavior, and environment across time. Throughout this book, we have explored the systems that shape brain longevity—neuroplasticity, metabolism, inflammation control, memory reinforcement, attentional stability, emotional regulation, social engagement, lifestyle architecture, and neural resilience. Each system contributes independently to cognitive function, yet their greatest protective power emerges when integrated consistently across daily living.

The brain does not age uniformly; it reflects the conditions it experiences. Neural decline often represents prolonged exposure to metabolic instability, inflammatory stress, sleep disruption, emotional overload, or cognitive underuse rather than unavoidable degeneration. When these pressures are reduced and supportive conditions are restored, the brain demonstrates remarkable capacity to stabilize and even recover function. Cognitive youth is therefore not preserved by resisting time but by maintaining biological compatibility with neural health.

A central principle emerging from this work is that cognitive longevity is dynamic rather than static. The brain continuously remodels itself in response to input. Every experience—movement, learning, nutrition, rest, connection, reflection—modifies neural circuitry. This ongoing plasticity means that cognitive trajectory remains modifiable throughout life. Even after periods of decline or neglect, improvement remains biologically possible when supportive inputs are reintroduced consistently.

Consistency outweighs intensity in neural preservation. Small, repeated behaviors shape brain physiology more powerfully than sporadic extremes. Stable sleep rhythms, regular cognitive challenge, balanced nutrition, physical movement, emotional regulation, and meaningful engagement cumulatively reinforce neural networks across decades. These patterns build reserve gradually, enabling the brain to tolerate aging-related pressures without losing function.

The concept of cognitive reserve reframes aging from inevitability to preparation. Brains enriched through learning, curiosity, and engagement develop dense, flexible networks capable of compensating for structural changes. Such brains maintain clarity and adaptability despite biological aging. Reserve is not inherited alone; it is constructed through lifelong interaction with environment and behavior.

Equally important is neural safety. The brain functions optimally when physiological and emotional environments signal stability rather than threat. Chronic stress, isolation, and overstimulation disrupt this safety, diverting neural resources toward survival responses. Restoration of calm, connection, and predictability allows higher cognitive networks to operate efficiently. Cognitive youth therefore depends on both stimulation and safety in balance.

Aging inevitably alters pace and processing speed, yet it need not erase capability. With preserved neural networks, individuals retain memory, reasoning, creativity, and identity across decades. Cognitive youth in later life often manifests not as youthful speed but as sustained clarity and adaptability. The goal of brain longevity is not resisting maturation but maintaining function through change.

Future neuroscience will likely expand tools for supporting brain health, but foundational principles will remain behavioral. Daily life conditions continue to shape neural physiology more than any isolated therapy. Individuals retain substantial agency over cognitive trajectory through sustained alignment with biological requirements for brain function.

Ultimately, cognitive youth represents continuity—the preservation of thought, memory, personality, and awareness across time. It allows individuals to remain mentally present within their lives, relationships, and experiences. This continuity defines quality of life more deeply than lifespan alone. Protecting the brain therefore protects the lived self.

The material in this book converges on a simple but powerful conclusion: the brain you inhabit later in life is built through the way you live earlier and continually. Every day contributes to neural structure and function. Cognitive longevity is not accidental; it is cultivated.

Daniel spoke without notes

Near his ninetieth birthday, Daniel still began mornings with quiet reading. The ritual had lasted decades. Tea, sunlight, pages turning slowly. Visitors often remarked on his clarity. Conversations with him carried depth and recall that surprised those half his age.

Daniel never considered himself exceptional. He had simply followed rhythms that felt natural—learning continually, walking daily, resting when needed, staying connected to others. He did not think of these as brain strategies. They were ways of living.

In his seventies, he had noticed peers withdrawing mentally. Complaints of forgetfulness, confusion, fatigue became common. Daniel listened with curiosity. His own mind felt steady, perhaps slower but not diminished. He wondered why trajectories differed so widely.

Only later did he understand that years of consistent engagement had built resilience quietly. His routines had nourished neural systems long before aging pressures appeared. When those pressures arrived, his brain had reserve to absorb them.

At eighty-five, he learned digital photography, fascinated by light and composition. Friends joked about starting new skills so late. Daniel simply enjoyed curiosity. The learning process energized him. He felt mentally alive, not preserving youth but expressing it.

On his ninetieth birthday, surrounded by family, Daniel spoke without notes. Stories flowed clearly—childhood scenes, lessons learned, humor intact. His memory did not feel miraculous; it felt continuous. He recognized faces, recalled moments, remained present.

Later that evening, sitting quietly, he reflected on a life still mentally accessible to him. Nothing had been lost abruptly. Time had passed, yet awareness remained connected to every stage. That continuity felt like his greatest fortune. Daniel understood then that cognitive youth was not youthfulness itself. It was the preservation of self across time. His mind had matured, adapted, and slowed gently without breaking. He remained himself fully.

His life illustrated the core message of this book: the brain responds to how it is lived with. Care, curiosity, movement, and connection accumulated into resilience. Aging revealed that accumulation rather than erasing it.

Daniel did not defeat time. He aligned with biology. And through that alignment, his cognitive presence endured into advanced age with grace.

www.ingramcontent.com/pod-product-compliance
Lightning Source LLC
LaVergne TN
LVHW022013200926
848481LV00007B/2374
* 9 7 9 8 2 9 5 6 7 1 3 1 9 *